PARKINSON DISEASE COOKBOOK

DR. NANCY GOLD

TABLE OF CONTENT

INTRODUCTION

Parkinson Disease

Parkinson's disease (PD), or simply Parkinson's, is a long-term degenerative disorder of the central nervous system that mainly affects the motor system. The symptoms usually emerge slowly, and as the disease worsens, non-motor symptoms become more common.

The most obvious early symptoms are tremor, rigidity, slowness of movement, and difficulty with walking. Cognitive and behavioral problems may also occur with depression, anxiety, and apathy occurring in many people with PD.

Parkinson's disease dementia becomes common in the advanced stages of the disease. Those with Parkinson's can also have problems with their sleep and sensory systems.

The motor symptoms of the disease result from the death of cells in the substantia nigra, a region of the midbrain, leading to a dopamine deficit.

The cause of this cell death is poorly understood, but involves the build-up of misfolded proteins into Lewy bodies in the neurons. Collectively, the main motor symptoms are also known as parkinsonism or a parkinsonian syndrome.

Classification

Parkinson's disease is the most common form of parkinsonism and is sometimes called "idiopathic parkinsonism", meaning parkinsonism with no identifiable cause.

It is sometimes referred to as a type of neurodegenerative disease called synucleinopathy due to an abnormal accumulation of the protein alpha-synuclein in the brain.

There are other "Parkinsons plus" syndromes that can have similar movement symptoms, but have a variety of associated symptoms. Some of these are also synucleinopathies. Lewy body dementia involves motor symptoms with early onset of cognitive dysfunction and hallucinations, with these often (though not necessarily) preceding the motor symptoms. Alternatively, multiple systems atrophy or MSA usually has early onset of autonomic dysfunction (such as orthostasis), and may have autonomic predominance, cerebellar symptom predominance, or Parkinsonian predominance.

Other "Parkinsons plus" syndromes involve tau, rather than alpha-synuclein. These include Progressive Supranuclear Palsy (PSP) and Corticobasal Syndrome (CBS).

PSP predominantly involves rigidity, early falls, bulbar symptoms, and vertical gaze restriction; it can also be associated with frontotemporal dementia symptoms.

CBS involves asymmetric parkinsonism, dystonia, alien limb, and myoclonic jerking. These unique presentation timelines and associated symptoms can help develop these similar movement disorders from idiopathic Parkinson disease.

What Does Parkinson's Do to the Brain?

Deep down in your brain, there's an area called the substantia nigra, which is in the basal ganglia. Some of its cells make dopamine, a chemical that carries messages around your brain. When you need to scratch an itch or kick a ball, dopamine quickly carries a message to the nerve cell that controls that movement.

When that system is working well, your body moves smoothly and evenly. But when you have Parkinson's, the cells of your substantia nigra start to die. There's no replacing them, so your dopamine levels drop and you can't fire off as many messages to control smooth body movements.

Early on, you won't notice anything different. But as more and more cells die, you reach a tipping point where you start to have symptoms.

That may not be until 80% of the cells are gone, which is why you can have Parkinson's for quite a while before you realize it.

How Does Parkinson's Affect the Body?

The telltale symptoms all have to do with the way you move. You usually notice problems like:

Rigid muscles. It can happen on just about any part of your body. Doctors sometimes mistake early Parkinson's for arthritis.

Slow movements. You may find that even simple acts, like buttoning a shirt, take much longer than usual.

Tremors. Your hands, arms, legs, lips, jaw, or tongue are shaky when you're not using them.

Walking and balance problems. You may notice your arms aren't swinging as freely when you walk or you can't take long steps, so you have to shuffle instead.

Parkinson's can also cause a range of other issues, from depression to bladder problems to acting out dreams. It may be a while before abnormal movements start.

PARKINSON'S DISEASE

CAUSES, SYMPTOMS,

DIAGNOSIS AND TREATMENTS

Parkinson's disease is a brain disorder that causes unintended or uncontrollable movements, such as shaking, stiffness, and difficulty with balance and coordination.

Symptoms usually begin gradually and worsen over time. As the disease progresses, people may have difficulty walking and talking. They may also have mental and behavioral changes, sleep problems, depression, memory difficulties, and fatigue.

Older woman and her caregiverWhile virtually anyone could be at risk for developing Parkinson's, some research studies suggest this disease affects more men than women. It's unclear why, but studies are underway to understand factors that may increase a person's risk.

One clear risk is age: Although most people with Parkinson's first develop the disease after age 60, about 5% to 10% experience onset before the age of 50. Early-onset forms of Parkinson's are often, but not always, inherited, and some forms have been linked to specific gene mutations.

What causes Parkinson's disease?

The most prominent signs and symptoms of Parkinson's disease occur when nerve cells in the basal ganglia, an area of the brain that controls movement, become impaired and/or die. Normally, these nerve cells, or neurons, produce an important brain chemical known as dopamine. When the neurons die or become impaired, they produce less dopamine, which causes the movement problems associated with the disease. Scientists still do not know what causes the neurons to die.

a computer generated graphic of the brain with labels pointing to the basal ganglia.

People with Parkinson's disease also lose the nerve endings that produce norepinephrine, the main chemical messenger of the sympathetic nervous system, which controls many functions of the body, such as heart rate and blood pressure.

The loss of norepinephrine might help explain some of the non-movement features of Parkinson's, such as fatigue, irregular blood pressure, decreased movement of food through the digestive tract, and sudden drop in blood pressure when a person stands up from a sitting or lying position.

Many brain cells of people with Parkinson's disease contain Lewy bodies, unusual clumps of the protein alpha-synuclein. Scientists are trying to better understand the normal and abnormal functions of alpha-synuclein and its relationship to genetic mutations that impact Parkinson's and Lewy body dementia. Some cases of Parkinson's disease appear to be hereditary, and a few cases can be traced to specific genetic mutations. While genetics is thought to play a role in Parkinson's, in most cases the disease does not seem to run in families. Many researchers now believe that Parkinson's results from a combination of genetic and environmental factors, such as exposure to toxins.

Symptoms of Parkinson's disease

Parkinson's has four main symptoms:

Tremor in hands, arms, legs, jaw, or head

Muscle stiffness, where muscle remains contracted for a long time

Slowness of movement

Impaired balance and coordination, sometimes leading to falls

Other symptoms may include:

Depression and other emotional changes

Difficulty swallowing, chewing, and speaking

Urinary problems or constipation

Skin problems

The symptoms of Parkinson's and the rate of progression differ among individuals. Early symptoms of this disease are subtle and occur gradually. For example, people may feel mild tremors or have difficulty getting out of a chair. They may notice that they speak too softly, or that their handwriting is slow and looks cramped or small.

Friends or family members may be the first to notice changes in someone with early Parkinson's. They may see that the person's face lacks expression and animation, or that the person does not move an arm or leg normally.

People with Parkinson's disease often develop a parkinsonian gait that includes a tendency to lean forward; take small, quick steps; and reduce swinging their arms. They also may have trouble initiating or continuing movement.

Symptoms often begin on one side of the body or even in one limb on one side of the body. As the disease progresses, it eventually affects both sides.

However, the symptoms may still be more severe on one side than on the other.

Many people with Parkinson's disease note that prior to experiencing stiffness and tremor, they had sleep problems, constipation, loss of smell, and restless legs. While some of these symptoms may also occur with normal aging, talk with your doctor if these symptoms worsen or begin to interfere with daily living.

Changes in cognition and Parkinson's disease

Some people with Parkinson's may experience changes in their cognitive function, including problems with memory, attention, and the ability to plan and accomplish tasks. Stress, depression, and some medications may also contribute to these changes in cognition.

Over time, as the disease progresses, some people may develop dementia and be diagnosed with Parkinson's dementia, a type of Lewy body dementia. People with Parkinson's dementia may have severe memory and thinking problems that affect daily living.

Talk with your doctor if you or a loved one is diagnosed with Parkinson's disease and is experiencing problems with thinking or memory.

Diagnosis of Parkinson's disease

There are currently no blood or laboratory tests to diagnose non-genetic cases of Parkinson's. Doctors usually diagnose the disease by taking a person's medical history and performing a neurological examination.

If symptoms improve after starting to take medication, it's another indicator that the person has Parkinson's.

A number of disorders can cause symptoms similar to those of Parkinson's disease. People with Parkinson's-like symptoms that result from other causes, such as multiple system atrophy and dementia with Lewy bodies, are sometimes said to have parkinsonism.

While these disorders initially may be misdiagnosed as Parkinson's, certain medical tests, as well as response to drug treatment, may help to better evaluate the cause. Many other diseases have similar features but require different treatments, so it is important to get an accurate diagnosis as soon as possible.

Treatments for Parkinson's disease

Although there is no cure for Parkinson's disease, medicines, surgical treatment, and other therapies can often relieve some symptoms.

Medicines for Parkinson's disease

Medicines can help treat the symptoms of Parkinson's by:

Increasing the level of dopamine in the brain

Having an effect on other brain chemicals, such as neurotransmitters, which transfer information between brain cells

Helping control non-movement symptoms

The main therapy for Parkinson's is levodopa. Nerve cells use levodopa to make dopamine to replenish the brain's dwindling supply. Usually, people take levodopa along with another medication called carbidopa.

Carbidopa prevents or reduces some of the side effects of levodopa therapy such as nausea, vomiting, low blood pressure, and restlessness and reduces the amount of levodopa needed to improve symptoms.

People living with Parkinson's disease should never stop taking levodopa without telling their doctor. Suddenly stopping the drug may have serious side effects, like being unable to move or having difficulty breathing.

The doctor may prescribe other medicines to treat Parkinson's symptoms, including:

Dopamine agonists to stimulate the production of dopamine in the brain Enzyme inhibitors (e.g., MAO-B inhibitors, COMT inhibitors) to increase the amount of dopamine by slowing down the enzymes that break down dopamine in the brain

Amantadine to help reduce involuntary movements

Anticholinergic drugs to reduce tremors and muscle rigidity

Deep brain stimulation

For people with Parkinson's disease who do not respond well to medications, the doctor may recommend deep brain stimulation. During a surgical procedure, a doctor implants electrodes into part of the brain and connects them to a small electrical device implanted in the chest. The device and electrodes painlessly stimulate specific areas in the brain that control movement in a way that may help stop many of the movement-related symptoms of Parkinson's, such as tremor, slowness of movement, and rigidity.

Other therapies

Other therapies that may help manage Parkinson's symptoms include:

Physical, occupational, and speech therapies, which may help with gait and voice disorders, tremors and rigidity, and decline in mental functions

A healthy diet to support overall wellness

Exercises to strengthen muscles and improve balance, flexibility, and coordination

Massage therapy to reduce tension

Yoga and tai chi to increase stretching and flexibility

Support for people living with Parkinson's disease

While the progression of Parkinson's is usually slow, eventually a person's daily routines may be affected. Activities such as working, taking care of a home, and participating in social activities with friends may become challenging.

Experiencing these changes can be difficult, but support groups can help people cope. These groups can provide information, advice, and connections to resources for those living with Parkinson's disease, their families, and caregivers.

The organizations listed below can help people find local support groups and other resources in their communities.

The 5 stages of parkinson disease

Stage one

Individuals experience mild symptoms that generally do not interfere with daily activities. Tremor and other movement symptoms occur on one side of the body only. They may also experience changes in posture, walking and facial expressions.

Stage two

Symptoms worsen, including tremor, rigidity and other movement symptoms on both sides of the body.

The person is still able to live alone, but daily tasks are more difficult and lengthier.

Stage three

This is considered mid-stage. Individuals experience loss of balance and slowness of movements. While still fully independent, these symptoms significantly impair activities such as dressing and eating. Falls are also more common by stage three.

Stage four

Symptoms are severe and limiting. Individuals may stand without help, but movement likely requires a walker. People in stage four require help with daily activities and are unable to live alone.

Stage five

Stiffness in the legs may make it impossible to stand or walk. The person requires a wheelchair or is bedridden. Around-the-clock nursing care is needed for all activities. The person may experience hallucinations and delusions.

Parkinson's diet

Parkinson's disease is a neurological condition that affects a person's movement. Certain dietary patterns are linked to a lower risk of Parkinson's. Also, for some people with this condition, making certain dietary changes may help control the symptoms.

Parkinson's disease can affect anyone. However, it affects around 50% more males than females.

Some common symptoms of Parkinson's include:

shaking

stiffness

difficulty with walking

balance issues

problems with coordination

The symptoms of Parkinson's tend to develop gradually over a period of several years. Early symptoms might include a slight tremor in one hand and a general feeling of stiffness in the body.

The National Institutes of Health (NIH) point out that, in the United States, around 50,000 people receive a diagnosis of Parkinson's each year.

Diet is one potential factor that may reduce the risk of Parkinson's or slow its progression.

This book will look at foods that may help a person reduce their Parkinson's symptoms. It will also look at foods that may make the symptoms worse.

Foods that may help Parkinson's

The following foods may be beneficial for slowing disease progression or for lowering the risk of Parkinson's disease.

Fish oil and omega-3 fatty acids

Some research suggests that fish oil may help slow the progressionTrusted Source of Parkinson's.

Studies suggest that omega-3 fats may help reduce nerve inflammation, improve neurotransmission, and slow neurodegenerationTrusted Source. Therefore, consuming more fatty fish rich in omega-3s or taking an omega-3 supplement may benefit people with Parkinson's.

Fish and seafood that contain high levels of omega-3 fatty acids include:

mackerel

salmon

herring

oysters

sardines

anchovies

Fish oil is a good source of omega-3 fatty acids, which have a number of other health benefits. It may also help improve cardiovascular healthTrusted Source and brain function and help slow the rate of cognitive decline.

In addition, to possibly offering direct benefits to those with Parkinson's, omega-3 fatty acids may also help reduce the riskTrusted Source of dementia and confusion more generally. These are also secondary symptoms of Parkinson's.

Fava beans

The most effective medication for Parkinson's is levodopa. Fava beans contain levodopa, so some people believe that they can help treat the symptoms of Parkinson's.

Fava beans may help people with Parkinson's, but it is important that people do not use them as an alternative to prescription treatments.

There has not been a lot of research into the efficacy of fava beans in slowing the progression of Parkinson's. However, one study does suggest that the consumption of fava beans may lead to a marked improvement in the motor performance of people with Parkinson's, without causing any side effects.

Foods containing nutrients that people may be deficient in

Some research suggests that people with Parkinson's often have certain nutrient deficiencies, including deficiencies in iron, vitamin B1, vitamin C, zinc, and vitamin D.

The above study points out that some of these deficiencies may be associated with neuroinflammation and neurodegeneration, which are key factors in Parkinson's.

Therefore, people with Parkinson's may wish to consume more of the following foods.

Foods containing iron

The following foods are good sources of iron:

liver

red meat

beans

nuts

Foods containing vitamin B1

The following foods are good sources of vitamin B1:

peas

bananas

oranges

nuts

wholegrain bread

Foods containing vitamin C

The following foods are good sources of vitamin C:

citrus fruits

peppers

strawberries

broccoli

potatoes

Foods containing zinc

The following foods are good sources of zinc:

meat

shellfish

bread

cereal products, such as wheat germ

Foods containing vitamin D

The following foods are good sources of vitamin D:

oily fish

red meat

egg yolks

certain fortified foods

Foods containing antioxidants

Free radicals are unstable molecules in the body. They are necessary for health. However, if there is an imbalance and there are more free radicals present than necessary, they can cause damage to fatty tissue, DNA, and proteins in the body.

The damage that these free radicals cause is known as oxidative stress. This is a condition that occurs when the amount of free radicals in the body is too high, which contributes to cellular damage. Some research has linked oxidative stress to the progression of Parkinson's.

Antioxidants keep free radicals in check, so following a diet high in antioxidants can help combat oxidative stress. Therefore, a person with Parkinson's may wish to consume antioxidant-rich foods in their diet.

Some good sources of antioxidants include:

blueberries, cranberries, grapes, cherries, strawberries, and raspberries

pecans, walnuts, and brazil nuts

spices such as turmeric

herbs such as parsley

cocoa powder and cacao products

broccoli, artichokes, spinach, and kale

citrus fruits

green tea

navy beans, black beans, and kidney beans

A healthy diet in general

While the above foods may be beneficial for people with Parkinson's, it is most important for people with Parkinson's to focus on their diet as a whole.

The Parkinson's Foundation suggest that people with Parkinson's follow these dietary tips:

Avoid fad diets and try to consume foods from all food groups.

Consume plenty of grains, vegetables, and fruits.

Limit sugar intake.

Reduce salt and sodium intake.

Consume foods that contain antioxidants, such as brightly colored and dark fruits and vegetables.

Follow a diet that is low in fat, saturated fat, and cholesterol.

Drink alcohol only in moderation.

Foods to avoid

There are a number of foods that may worsen the symptoms of Parkinson's disease or speed up the progression of the condition. These foods include the following.

Processed foods

Some studies suggest that eating a "Western-style" diet may be linked with symptom severity in Parkinson's.

This type of diet is high in processed foods. Some examples of processed foods include:

canned foods

sodas

breakfast cereals

chips

bacon

ready meals

candy

cakes

One study suggests that several of these items, including canned foods and sodas, may be associated with "more rapid Parkinson's progression."

Also, the researcher behind another studyTrusted Source points out that eating a lot of processed foods "contributes to increased intestinal permeability and dysbiosis due to an overgrowth of gram-negative bacteria."

They add that there seems to be a "positive correlation" between this increased intestinal permeability and the severity of Parkinson's symptoms.

The researcher suggests that this may be due to the neurotoxic molecules produced by these bacteria passing into the bloodstream and causing gut-related symptoms that extend to the esophagus (food pipe) and oropharyngeal cavity.

Symptoms such as difficulty swallowing and problems with speech and smell are common in Parkinson's.

Given that processed foods may be linked with symptom severity in Parkinson's, people with this condition may wish to avoid them.

Certain dairy foods

Some research suggests that dairy products may be linked with a higher risk of Parkinson's. For example, one studyTrusted Source suggests that the consumption of skim and low fat milk may be associated with an increased risk of the condition.

Another study adds that yogurt and cheese consumption may be associated with faster disease progression in Parkinson's.

Therefore, a person with Parkinson's may wish to avoid consuming large quantities of these dairy products.

Foods containing saturated fat and cholesterol

Some studies suggest that dietary fat intake may increase the risk of Parkinson's.

Although having a higher intake of cholesterol can elevate a person's Parkinson's risk, having a higher intake of polyunsaturated fatty acids may reduce the risk.

Therefore, a person with Parkinson's may wish to reduce their intake of cholesterol to help control the symptoms of the condition. They may also wish to reduce the amount of saturated fat in their diet. However, further studies are required to explore the link between dietary fat and Parkinson's.

Foods that are hard to chew

Many people with Parkinson's have difficulty with chewing and swallowing foods. A person needs medical help if this is the case.

A speech and language therapist may be able to help a person overcome this issue.

However, if a person is finding certain foods hard to chew and swallow, they may wish to avoid these foods.

Such foods include:

hard foods

dry, crumbly foods

tough or chewy meats

If a person does wish to eat chewy meats, they could try using gravy or sauce to soften them and make eating easier.

They could also try chopping meat into smaller pieces or incorporating meat into casseroles, which can make it more tender.

Having a drink with a meal can also make chewing and swallowing easier.

PARKINSON DISEASE RECIPES

SNACKS

1. Apple Crumble Squares

Equipment:

Measuring spoons

9 x 13 in. (3.5 L) baking pan

Whisk

Parchment paper

Knife

Cutting board

Rubber spatula

Toothpicks

Ingredients:

1½ cups (375 mL) All-purpose flour

1 tsp (5 mL) Baking powder

1 tsp (5 mL) Cinnamon

½ tsp (2 mL) Salt

½ cup (125 mL) Sugar

½ cup (125 mL) Brown sugar, loosely packed

2 each Eggs

⅓ cup (75 mL) Vegetable oil

1 tsp (5 mL) Vanilla extract

4 cups (1 L) McIntosh apples, unpeeled, cored and ½ in. diced

Method:

Preheat oven to 350°F (180°C). Line a 9 x 13 in. (3.5 L) pan with parchment paper and set aside.

Sift flour, baking powder, cinnamon, and salt together in a medium bowl and set aside.

In a large bowl, whisk together sugar, brown sugar, eggs, vegetable oil and vanilla extract until smooth.

Mix dry ingredients into wet ingredients until just incorporated.

Fold apples into the batter and spread evenly with spatula onto lined baking pan.

To prepare topping, place the ingredients in a medium bowl and gently rub together with fingertips until crumbly.

Top batter with crumb topping, and bake for 45-55 minutes. Cake is ready when an inserted toothpick comes out clean.

2. Fruit Bars

Equipment:

8 in. (2L) square pan

Parchment paper

Small sauce pan

Mixing bowls

Measuring cups

Knife

Cutting board

Rubber spatula

Ingredients:

Base:

¾ cup (175 mL) Rolled oats, large flakes

½ cup (125 mL) All-purpose flour

½ cup (125 mL) Tapioca flour

½ cup (125 mL) Brown sugar, loosely packed

½ cup (125 mL) Dried shredded coconut, unsweetened

½ cup (125 mL) Dried apricots, finely chopped

½ cup (125 mL) Dried cranberries, roughly chopped

½ cup (125 mL) Raisins

½ cup (125 mL) Butter, softened

Topping:

½ cup (125 mL) Semi-sweet chocolate

Method:

Preheat oven to 350°F (180°C). Line an 8 in. (2L) square pan with parchment paper and set aside.

In a medium bowl, blend all the dry ingredients together with fingers. Add mixture to softened butter and continue mixing with fingers until crumbly.

Spread into the lined baking pan and pat down firmly.

Bake for 15 to 20 minutes. You will know bars are ready when they are golden brown on the top.

Remove from oven and let cool to room temperature for 15 minutes. Refrigerate for 15 minutes until it is cold.

Melt chocolate in microwave and let cool to room temperature.

Spread onto cold fruit bars with a rubber spatula and return to refrigerator until chocolate is set. Cut into 24 bars.

3. Banana Berry Smoothies

Equipment:

Blender

Measuring cups

Measuring spoons

Knife

Ingredients:

2 cups (500 mL) Orange juice

2 each Banana, cut in half

2 cups (500 mL) Blueberries, frozen

1 cup (250 mL) Strawberries, frozen

2 tbsp (30 mL) Honey

Method:

In a blender, purée all ingredients until smooth.

Pour into an airtight container and keep refrigerated.

4. Chocolate & Orange Date Cake

Equipment:

Knife

8 in. (2L) square pan

Small sauce pot

Wooden spoon

Measuring cups

Measuring spoons

Orange zester

Ingredients:

1¾ cup (425 mL) Dried dates, pitted and chopped

⅓ cup (75 mL) Maple syrup

1 each Orange zest

¾ cup (175 mL) Water

½ cup (125 mL) Butter, room temperature

½ cup (125 mL) Sugar

1½ cup (375 mL) Tapioca flour

½ cup (125 mL) Cocoa powder

¼ tsp (1 mL) Baking soda

Pinch Salt

3 tbsp (45 mL) Almond milk

Method:

Preheat oven to 350°F (180°C). Line 8 in. (2L) square pan with parchment paper and set aside.

In a sauce pan combine the dates, maple syrup, orange zest and water.

Simmer until mixture thickens to a jam consistency, approximately 15 minutes.

In a large mixing bowl, cream together butter and sugar and set aside.

In a separate bowl combine the tapioca flour, cocoa powder, baking soda and salt. Stir to combine.

Mix dry ingredients into the butter and sugar. Stir in the thickened cooked dates and almond milk.

Spread mixture into lined pan and bake for 30 to 35 minutes. Let cool completely before slicing.

5. Pina Colada Cupcakes

Equipment:

Mixing bowls

Measuring cups

Measuring spoons

Muffin pan

Medium cupcake liners

Strainer

Whisk

Knife

Rubber spatula

Toothpicks

Ingredients:

Cupcakes:

1¼ cup (300 mL) All-purpose flour

¼ cup (60 mL) Dried shredded coconut, unsweetened

½ cup (125 mL) Sugar

½ tsp (2 mL) Baking powder

½ tsp (2 mL) Baking soda

¼ tsp (1 mL) Salt

½ cup (125 mL) Coconut milk

¾ cup (175 mL) Crushed pineapple, canned and well drained. Reserve juice.

½ cup (125 mL) Pineapple juice, from drained pineapple

¼ cup (60 mL) Vegetable oil

½ tsp (2 mL) Vanilla extract

Coconut Glaze:

1 cup (250 mL) Confectioner's sugar

1 tbsp (15 mL) Butter, softened

3 tbsp (45 mL) Coconut milk

1 tsp (5 mL) Vanilla extract

Method:

Cupcakes:

Preheat oven to 350°F (180°C). Line cupcake pan with liners and set aside.

In a large bowl, combine flour, shredded coconut, sugar, baking powder, baking soda and salt.

In a separate bowl, whisk together coconut milk, pineapple juice, vegetable oil and vanilla extract.

Add wet ingredients to dry ingredients and stir to combine.

Lastly, gently stir in crushed pineapple until just incorporated.

Using an ice cream scoop, divide batter into lined pan.

Bake for 25-30 minutes or until inserted toothpick comes out clean. Allow to cool in pan for 5 minutes, and then transfer to a wire rack to cool completely.

Coconut Glaze:

Whisk confectioner's sugar, butter, coconut milk and vanilla extract together until combined. About 30 seconds.

When cupcakes are completely cooled, frost with 2 tsp (10 mL) of icing each.

6. Strawberry Mango Smoothie

Equipment:

Blender

Knife

Measuring cups

Measuring spoons

Ingredients:

2 cups (500 mL) Almond milk

1 each Banana, cut in half

2 cups (500 mL) Mango, frozen

2 cups (500 mL) Strawberries, frozen

2 tbsp (30 mL) Honey

Method:

In a blender, purée all ingredients until smooth.

Pour into an airtight container and keep refrigerated.

BREAKFAST

7. Blueberry Pancakes

Equipment:

Mixing bowls

Whisk

Non-stick skillet

Measuring cups

Measuring spoons

Lemon zester

Pastry brush

Spatula

Ingredients:

1 cup (250 mL) Gluten free all-purpose flour

2 tsp (10 mL) Baking powder

1 tsp (5 mL) Xanthan gum (if your gluten free flour already contains xanthan gum, omit from recipe)

2 tbsp (30 mL) Sugar

1 each Egg

1 cup (250 mL) Almond milk

2 tbsp (30 mL) Vegetable oil

1 tsp (5 mL) Vanilla extract

1 each Lemon, zest and juice

1 cup (250 mL) Blueberries, fresh

2 tbsp (30 mL) Butter, melted

Method:

In a medium bowl, whisk together the flour, baking powder, xanthan gum and sugar.

In a small bowl, mix egg, almond milk, vegetable oil, vanilla, lemon zest and juice.

Add wet ingredients to dry ingredients all at once and whisk until combined. Stir in fresh blueberries

Heat non-stick skillet on medium-high heat and brush pan with a little melted butter.

Pour ¼ cup (60 mL) of batter onto frying pan and cook until bottom is brown and bubbles appear on top.

Flip pancake and cook for another 1-2 minutes until cooked through.

8. Roasted Potatoes & Tomatoes

Equipment:

Knife

Cutting board

Baking tray

Parchment paper

Large pot

Strainer

Mixing bowls

Measuring spoons

Wooden spoon

Spatula

Ingredients:

1 tbsp (15 mL) Baking soda/li>

3 each Russet potatoes, ½ in. diced

1 tbsp (15 mL) Paprika

1 tsp (5 mL) Salt

1 tbsp (15 mL) Olive oil

1 each Red pepper, thinly sliced

1 each Red onion, thinly sliced

1 pint Cherry tomatoes, cut in half

3 sprigs Basil leaves, chopped

To taste Salt and pepper

Method:

Preheat oven to 475°F (240°C). Line a large baking tray with parchment paper and set aside.

Bring a large pot of water to boil. Add baking soda and potatoes to the boiling water.

Allow water to return to a boil and cook for 2 minutes.

Drain potatoes and transfer to a mixing bowl. Add paprika, salt and 1 tbsp (15 mL) olive oil. Mix until potatoes are evenly coated.

Toss potatoes with peppers and onions and place onto the prepared baking tray.

Bake for 10 minutes, flip potatoes using a spatula and return to oven for another 15 minutes

You will know that they are finished when you can stick a knife into the potatoes very easily. Season with salt and pepper.

Mix tomatoes and basil together with remaining olive oil. Season with salt and pepper and serve with roasted potatoes.

9. Zucchini & Chocolate Cranberry Muffins

muffins

Equipment:

Muffin tin

Paper muffin liners

Grater

Mixing bowls

Wooden spoon

Measuring cups

Measuring spoons

Toothpicks

Ingredients:

1 ½ cup (375 mL) Gluten free all-purpose flour

2 tsp (10 mL) Baking powder

½ tsp (2 mL) Baking soda

¾ tsp (4 mL) Xanthan gum (If your flour contains xanthan gum, omit this extra xanthan gum.)

¼ cup (60 mL) Brown sugar

¾ cup (175 mL) Almond milk

2 tbsp (30 mL) Honey

1 each Egg

1 tsp (5 mL) Vanilla extract

1 cup (250 mL) Zucchini, finely grated

1 cup (250 mL) Dried cranberries

½ cup (125 mL) Dark chocolate chips

Method:

Preheat oven to 375°F (190°C). Line muffin tins with paper muffin cups and set aside.

Melt butter in microwave and set aside to cool.

In a large bowl, combine flour, baking powder, baking soda, xanthan gum and sugar mix thoroughly.

In a separate bowl, mix the almond milk, egg, cooled butter and vanilla extract.

Mix wet ingredients into the dry ingredients until smooth.

Gently mix in the grated zucchini, cranberry, dark chocolate chips until just incorporated. Batter should be lumpy.

Divide the batter evenly among the muffin cups.

Bake for 25-30 minutes, until a toothpick inserted into the centre comes out clean, and muffins are lightly browned.

LUNCH

10. Ginger & Veg Stir-Fry

Equipment:

Large pot

Large wok or large sauté pan

Strainer

Mixing bowls

Knife

Cutting board

Grater

Measuring cups

Measuring spoons

Wooden spoon

Tongs

Ingredients:

125 g (⅓ pkg) Rice noodles, wide

1 tbsp (15 mL) Cornstarch

¼ cup (60 mL) Vegetable oil

2 cups (500 mL) Broccoli florets, bite-sized

1 each Carrot, thinly sliced half-moon shape

1 pkg (226 g) Mushrooms, quartered

1 each Red pepper, thinly sliced

1 each Yellow pepper, thinly sliced

½ cup (125 mL) Snow peas, stem removed

1 each Onion, sliced

1 clove Garlic, grated

2 tsp (10 mL) Ginger, grated

3 tbsp (45 mL) Soy sauce, light

3 tbsp (45 mL) Water

½ tsp (2 mL) Salt

Method:

Bring a large pot of water to a boil and remove from heat. Put rice noodles into pot and soak until they are al dente (approximately 20-25 minutes). Check noodles periodically to make sure they do not become too soft.

When noodles are al dente, rinse with cold water and drain. Set aside.

In a large bowl, mix cornstarch and 2 tbsp (30 mL) of vegetable oil together until cornstarch is dissolved.

Toss broccoli, carrots, mushrooms, red pepper, yellow pepper and snow peas in cornstarch mixture to coat.

Heat the remaining oil, 2 tbsp (30 mL), in a large wok over medium high heat. Sauté onions, garlic and ginger with oil.

Add vegetables and cook for 2 minutes, stirring constantly to prevent burning.

Mix soy sauce, water and salt together and add to the wok.

Add soaked rice noodles and gently stir fry until vegetables are cooked and tender. Do not over mix.

11. Onion Gravy

Equipment:

Knife

Cutting board

Small saucepan

Wooden spoon

Measuring cups

Measuring spoons

Immersion hand blender

Ingredients:

1 tbsp (15 mL) Butter

1 tbsp (15 mL) Vegetable oil

2 each Onions, finely chopped

1 tsp (5 mL) Sugar

1 tsp (5 mL) Red wine vinegar

2 cups (500 mL) Vegetable stock

1 tbsp (15 mL) Dijon mustard

1 pinch Black pepper

To taste Salt

Method:

In a small sauce pot on low heat, melt butter and add the vegetable oil.

Add onions and cook on low heat until they are browned and soft. Approximately 20 minutes.

Add sugar and cook for 2 minutes. Stir in vinegar and stock and cook for an additional 10 minutes or until gravy has reduced by half.

Stir in mustard and pepper. Season to taste with salt.

Remove from heat and using a hand blender, blend until smooth.

12. Potato & Mushroom Pie

Equipment:

Potato peeler

Knife

Cutting board

Measuring cups

Measuring spoons

Grater

Pastry brush

Medium pot

Strainer

Large skillet

Wooden spoon

Non-stick muffin tin

Ingredients:

½ each Potato, peeled and parboiled, ½ in. diced

2 tbsp (30 mL) Vegetable oil

1 each Onion, ½ in. diced

1 clove Garlic, minced

½ tsp (2 mL) Rosemary, dried

1 tsp (5 mL) Thyme, dried

1 cup (250 mL) Mushrooms, ½ in. diced

½ each Sweet potato, peeled and coarsely grated

1 tbsp (15 mL) Lemon juice

To taste Salt and pepper

3 tbsp (45 mL) Butter

4 sheets Phyllo pastry

Method:

Preheat oven to 375°F (190°C).

In a medium pot, bring 2 cups (500 mL) of water to a boil and add diced potatoes.

Return to a boil and cook for 2 minutes. Drain potatoes, run under cold water and set aside.

Heat oil in large skillet and add onions, garlic, rosemary and thyme. Cook until onions become translucent and add potatoes.

When potatoes are golden, stir in the grated sweet potato, 1 tbsp (15 mL) of butter and mushrooms. Cook until mushrooms are tender and add lemon juice.

Season with salt and pepper and allow filling to cool.

Melt the remaining butter and set aside.

Lay 1 sheet of phyllo dough onto a clean cutting board and brush the entire surface with melted butter. Place another sheet of phyllo dough on top. Cut into 6 equal pieces. Repeat this step with remaining 2 sheets of dough.

Line a standard size non-stick muffin tin with the phyllo squares allowing sides to hang over.

Place approximately ⅓ cup (75 mL) of filling into each muffin cup and fold hanging dough over to seal the pies.

Brush with remaining butter and bake for 15 minutes or until the pies are flaky and golden brown.

Gently remove from muffin tins and allow to cool on wire rack.

13. Spicy Ketchup

Equipment:

Knife

Cutting board

Small pot

Measuring cups

Measuring spoons

Wooden spoon

Immersion hand blender

Ingredients:

2 tbsp (30 mL) Vegetable oil

1 each Onion, diced

4 cloves Garlic, minced

1 each Red bell pepper, diced

½ cup (125 mL) Tomato paste

1 tsp (5 mL) Chili flakes, dried

2 tbsp (30 mL) Red wine vinegar

¼ cup (60 mL) Brown sugar, packed

2 tsp (10 mL) Salt

1 tsp (5 mL) Black pepper

Method:

Heat oil in a small pot. Cook onions, garlic and red bell pepper until onions are caramelized on a low heat for 10 minutes, stirring often to prevent burning.

Stir in tomato paste, chili flakes, vinegar and sugar. Cook for an additional 10 minutes.

Remove pot from stove and purée using a hand blender.

Season with salt and pepper

14. Veg Medley Stew

Equipment:

Cutting board

Knife

Measuring cups

Measuring spoons

Large stock pot

Large saute pan

Hand held immersion blender

Can opener

Ingredients:

¼ cup (60 mL) Butter

1 each Onion, diced

3 each Garlic, minced

1 tsp (5 mL) Thyme, dried

1 tbsp (15 mL) Tomato paste

½ each Cauliflower, roughly chopped

3 cups (750 mL) Vegetable broth, low sodium

2 each Carrot, diced

1 each Red bell pepper, diced

2 each Zucchini, diced

1 can (796 mL) Diced canned tomatoes, with juices

1 tsp (5 mL) Salt

¼ tsp (1 mL) Black pepper

Method:

In a large stockpot, heat 2 tbsp (30 mL) of butter. Add onions, garlic, tomato paste and thyme. Cook over a low heat, stirring occasionally, until onions are transparent.

Add in cauliflower and 2 cups (500 mL) of stock. Bring to a boil and cook for approximately 5 minutes, until cauliflower is soft. Purée with hand blender until smooth.

Heat remaining 2 tbsp (30 mL) of butter in a large sauté pan and add carrots. Cook for 2 minutes and add red bell pepper. Cook until carrots and peppers are caramelized.

Stir carrots and peppers into cauliflower purée along with zucchini and diced tomatoes. Bring to a boil.

Add remaining stock and salt and pepper. Return to a boil and reduce to a simmer.

Cook for 20 minutes uncovered on a medium heat until stew has thickened. Season to taste.

DINNER

15. Salmon Fish Cakes

Equipment:

Mixing bowls

Knife

Cutting boards

Measuring cups

Measuring spoons

Can opener

Lemon zester

Spatula

Non-stick frying pan

Thermometer

Ingredients:

4 each Green onion, chopped

1 tbsp (15 mL) Dried dill

¼ tsp (1 mL) Salt

¼ tsp (1 mL) Black pepper

½ tsp (2 mL) Cayenne pepper (optional)

1 tsp (5 mL) Onion powder

1 each Lemon, zest and juice

1 each Egg

1 can (540 mL) Black beans, drained and rinsed

3 -213g cans Salmon, drained

½ cup (125 mL) All-purpose flour

¼ cup (60 mL) Vegetable oil

Method:

Combine green onion, dill, salt, black pepper, cayenne pepper, onion powder, lemon zest and juice, and egg in a medium bowl. Mix until well combined.

Using a fork, slightly mash beans in a small bowl and add to egg mixture.

Flake salmon into large pieces with a fork. Incorporate into bean and egg mixture. Add in ¼ cup (60 mL) flour and stir until combined.

Form into 8 cakes. Approximately ½ cup (125 mL) - ¾ cup (175 mL) of the mixture for each cake. Gently press together to hold and dust cakes with remaining flour.

Heat half the vegetable oil, 2 tbsp (30 mL) in fry pan over medium heat.

Bake for 10 minutes, flip potatoes using a spatula and return to oven for another 15 minutes

Place fish cakes in heated pan and cook for 4 minutes. Gently flip and cook for an additional 5 minutes or until the internal temperature reaches 160°F (71°C).

16. Veg Chili

Equipment:

Cutting board

Knife

Measuring cups

Measuring spoons

Wooden spoon

Can opener

Large pot

Ingredients:

1 each Onion, chopped

4 cloves Garlic, minced

1 tbsp (15 mL) Vegetable oil

1 can (540 mL) Bean medley, canned, rinsed

1 can (796 mL) Diced canned tomatoes, with juices

1 cup (250 mL) Corn, frozen

1 each Lime, juiced

2 tbsp (30 mL) Chili powder

1 each Jalapeño pepper, seeded, diced (optional)

2 tsp (10 mL) Paprika powder

1 tsp (5 mL) Salt

2 cups (500 mL) Tomato juice

1 ½ cups (375 mL) Textured vegetable protein

4 pieces Green onion, chopped

Method:

In a large pot, sauté the onions and garlic in vegetable oil until translucent.

Add beans, tomatoes, corn, lime juice, chili powder, jalapeño, paprika, salt and tomato juice. Mix thoroughly.

Cover pot and bring to a boil. Stir and reduce heat to a simmer.

Simmer while covered for about 20 minutes

Stir in textured vegetable protein and allow to cook for 3 – 5 more minutes. Season to taste. An additional ½ cup (125 mL) of water can be added if chili is too thick.

Stir in green onion. Season to taste.

17. Tartar Sauce

Equipment:

Small bowl

Knife

Cutting boards

Measuring cups

Measuring spoons

Ingredients:

¾ cup (175 mL) Mayonnaise

¼ cup (60 mL) Relish

1 tbsp (15 mL) Lemon juice

2 tbsp (30 mL) Green onion, chopped

¼ tsp (1 mL) Cayenne pepper (optional)

1 tsp (5 mL) Onion powder

1 each Lemon, zest and juice

1 each Egg

1 can (540 mL) Black beans, drained and rinsed

3 -213g cans Salmon, drained

½ cup (125 mL) All-purpose flour

¼ cup (60 mL) Vegetable oil

Method:

Combine all ingredients and mix well. Refrigerate in an airtight container until ready to serve.

18. Southwestern-style Chicken & Quinoa

Equipment:

Shallow baking dish

Medium pot

Fine mesh sieve

Tongs

Knife

Cutting board

Measuring cups

Measuring spoons

Wooden spoon

chicken quinoa nutrition

Ingredients:

4 each Chicken breasts, boneless and skinless

¾ tsp (4 mL) Salt

¼ tsp (1 mL) Black pepper

Pinch Paprika

1 tbsp (15 mL) Garlic powder

⅓ cup (75 mL) Lime juice, reserve 2 tbsp (30mL) for dressing

2 tbsp (30 mL) Olive oil, reserve 1 tbsp (15 mL) for dressing

1 cup (250 mL) Quinoa

½ cup (125 mL) Monterey Jack cheese, grated

4 each Green onion, chopped

¾ cup (175 mL) Corn, canned and drained

¾ cup (175 mL) Black beans, canned and drained

2 each Plum tomatoes, seeded, ½ in. diced

Method:

Preheat oven to 350°F (180°C).

Season chicken breast with salt, black pepper, paprika, garlic powder, 3 tbsp (45 mL) lime juice and 1 tbsp (15 mL) olive oil. Transfer to baking dish and place in preheated oven.

Rinse quinoa under running water for 3 minutes using a fine mesh sieve.

Cook quinoa according to package instructions. Once quinoa is cooked let rest, uncovered.

After 15 minutes of cooking, turn over chicken and continue to cook for an additional 10 minutes.

After 10 minutes, sprinkle chicken breasts with grated cheese and return to oven for an additional 3 minutes, or until cheese is melted. Remove from oven and cut into ½ in. slices.

Add ½ cup (125 mL) green onions, corn, black beans, and tomatoes to cooked quinoa.

Drizzle remaining 2 tbsp (30 mL) lime juice and 1 tbsp (15 mL) olive oil over quinoa. Season to taste with salt and toss to coat. Use remaining green onions as a garnish.

OTHERS

19. Mushroom and kidney bean pattie

Ingredients

1 medium sweet potato

2 large Portobello/Field mushrooms

Extra virgin olive oil

1 cup of cooked kidney beans

1 small carrot, roughly chopped

1/4 medium onion, roughly chopped

1 bunch fresh coriander, roughly chopped

Breadcrumbs

1 teaspoon fresh chili (optional)

1 teaspoon ground cumin

1 egg

Salad to serve (sliced tomato, lettuce leaves)

Method

Peel and cut the sweet potato into battens or chips – 2cm x 8cm. Place on a baking tray with non-stick paper.

Remove mushroom stalks, place on the same baking tray and drizzle with extra virgin olive oil.

Roast in a 200ºC (392ºF) oven for 20 minutes, or until mushrooms and sweet potato are cooked.

In a food processor combine kidney beans, carrot, onion, coriander, breadcrumbs and spices. Process to a rough paste. Transfer to a bowl and mix through the egg. Form into 2 patties.

Fry the patties in extra virgin olive oil until warmed through and browned on the outside.

To assemble, place the salad on the bottom of the plate, then the patty, your favourite sauce or chutney and top with the roasted mushroom.

Serve with the sweet potato chips on the side

20. Lentil and Vegetable Penne pasta

Ingredients

2 tablespoons extra virgin olive oil

3 small carrots, peeled, finely chopped

3 celery sticks, finely chopped

2 garlic cloves, thinly chopped

1 large brown onion, coarsely chopped

1 small red capsicum, finely chopped

10-12 button mushrooms, thinly chopped

225 grams cooked brown lentils

150 grams Passata

500 grams No added sugar pasta sauce

500 grams High fibre pasta – Penne

Method

Heat the extra virgin olive oil in a large heavy-based saucepan over medium heat.

Add celery, carrot, onion, garlic and cook until just tender.

Add lentils, capsicum and mushrooms and cook, until just tender.

Add Passata and pasta sauce, bring to the boil.

Reduce heat to medium-low and simmer for 20 minutes.

Meanwhile, bring a large pot of water to the boil over high heat. Add the penne pasta and cook, stirring often, for 10-12 mins or until tender. Drain.

Divide penne among serving bowls. Spoon over the sauce. Serve.

21. Creamy spinach sweet potato noodles with cashew sauce

This recipe caught my eye for people with Parkinson's. The sweet potato has been used in a fun way in this recipe which I love. Sweet potatoes are a good source of potassium and the antioxidants beta carotene and vitamin C as well as being high in fibre! Eating an adequate amount of fibre is one strategy to help manage and prevent constipation. Sweet potatoes also have a lower glycaemic index (GI) than regular potatoes and as you can see in this recipe are quite a versatile ingredient.

I also love how they have used cashews as part of this recipe! Cashews are a powerhouse of vitamins, minerals and other beneficial nutrients including the antioxidants lutein and zeaxanthin. Cashews are also rich in healthy fats and have a lovely buttery taste. And like sweet potato, cashews are also a very versatile ingredient.

Spinach is a green leafy vegetable that is such an easy ingredient to cook with and contains antioxidants which fight oxidative stress and help reduce the damage it causes.

To learn how to make Creamy spinach sweet potato noodles with cashew sauce be sure to check out the full details at Pinch of Yum.

22. Egg and vegetable muffins

Ingredients

4 eggs

15-20 spinach leaves, roughly chopped

¼ cup red capsicum, finely diced

¼ cup corn cornels (cooked)

6 cherry tomatoes (cut into quarters)

Method

Preheat the oven to 190°C/375°F.

Grease a 6-cup muffin tin or use paper cupcake cases.

Crack the eggs into a bowl and whisk together with a fork.

Add the capsicum, spinach, tomato and corn to the whisked eggs and stir.

Pour the egg mixture into the greased 6-cup muffin tin or paper cupcake cases.

Bake for 10-12 minutes or until eggs are set.

Allow to cool for 5 minutes before removing from muffin tin.

23. Beetroot and cashew puree

Ingredients

250 grams fresh Beetroot

60 grams unsalted Cashews

Extra virgin Olive Oil

Salt

Pepper

Equipment

Steamer

Stick blender with chopper attachment or a food processor

Sieve

Spoon

Method

Place whole beetroots into the bottom level of a bench top or cooktop steamer. Place cashews in the steaming basket above and cook until beetroot is tender.

Remove beetroot skins and place into the stick blender chopper/food processor along with the steamed cashews, salt and pepper & a drizzle of olive oil then blitz until smooth. Note— when blitzing, stop regularly to scrape down the sides of the processor or chopping attachment, drizzle more olive oil if mixture appears too dry.

Pass mixture through a sieve to ensure all hard, grainy particles are removed.

Using a touch of lemon infused olive oil works very well in this recipe if you have it available.

24. Roast pumpkin puree

Ingredients

500 grams butternut pumpkin

Extra virgin olive oil

Salt

Pepper

Equipment

Baking Dish

Stick blender

Jug or beaker

Method

Chop pumpkin, removing skin and seeds, and place in a baking dish.

Drizzle with extra virgin olive oil, sprinkle of salt and pepper and place into the oven.

Once tender remove from the oven and transfer into a jug/beaker.

Use stick blender to puree until smooth.

25. Carrot & Miso Soup with Silken Tofu

Ingredients

1 kg Carrots Peeled & Chopped

1 large Onion Diced

1.5 tsp Grated Fresh Ginger

3 cloves Garlic Crushed

1 litre Vegetable Stock

4 tbsp White Miso

200gm Silken Tofu

2 tbsp Sesame Oil

Salt

Pepper

Coconut cream & additional sesame oil for garnishing (or extra virgin olive oil)

Equipment

Blender or Stick Blender

Method

Sauté onions, garlic, ginger and carrots in sesame oil until onions are translucent. Add in vegetable stock, cover and simmer for 30 minutes stirring occasionally.

Add in white miso and silken tofu and blend using your modification tool of choice, adding more stock or water as needed (or alternatively coconut cream.) Add salt and pepper to taste.

Note – if requiring thickened fluids add in medically prescribed thickening agent during step 2.

Ladle into serving bowls and serve with a drizzle of sesame or extra virgin olive oil and a touch of coconut cream.

26. Chocolate smoothie recipes

Ingredients

150 ml unsweetened almond milk

½ avocado

4 fresh strawberries

1 teaspoon raw cacao powder

1½ teaspoon natvia (natural sweetener)

Ice to serve

Method

Combine almond milk, avocado flesh, strawberries, cacao and natvia in a blender.

Blend until smooth.

Serve in a glass with ice.

27. Berry smoothie with blueberries & strawberries

Ingredients

200 ml coconut water

1/2 cup strawberries

1/2 cup blueberries

1/2 cup coconut yoghurt

METHOD

In a blender, combine all ingredients and blend until smooth.

Serve in a glass.

28. Banana Oat and Cinnamon Smoothie

Ingredients

1 medium banana

250 ml oat milk

½ teaspoon ground cinnamon

½ teaspoon honey (optional)

Method

Peel the banana and break into pieces and add to the blender. Then add oat milk, cinnamon and honey if desired.

Blend until smooth.

Serve in a glass.

29. Mango Smothie

SMOOTHIE INGREDIENTS

1 medium Mango

170 ml coconut milk

100 ml coconut water

5-10 ice cubes (optional)

Method

Peel the mango and slice the flesh and add to the blender. Then add coconut milk, coconut water and ice if desired.

Blend until smooth.

Serve in a glass.

30. Chocolate avocado mousse

Ingredients

2 large avocados

3 tbsp honey

1 tsp vanilla bean extract

40 grams cocoa powder

Method

Place avocado flesh into a food processor with the honey, vanilla bean extract and cacao powder.

Blend/process until silky and smooth.

Transfer into chosen serving dish/es and refrigerate for at least 1 hour before serving.

CONCLUSION

There is still no cure for Parkinsons disease but there are Parkinsons disease treatments available today to reduce the severity of its symptoms.

Doctors generally advise patients to have a combination of Parkinsons disease treatments such as medications coupled with therapy.

Physical therapy is necessary because it enables the patient to retain his mobility and control over his muscles in spite of the usual tremors and other physical symptoms of Parkinsons disease. Speech therapy is, on the other hand, also necessary to combat difficulties with speaking and swallowing, two of the most well-known symptoms of the disease.

Different medications are used for treating Parkinsons disease. Over time, you might be asked to change your medication as it loses its effectiveness or increase its dosage.

Because of this, it's extremely crucial that you do not cease consulting with your doctor in a regular basis. Medications used for treating Parkinsons disease include Coenzyme Q10, amantadine, anticholigernics, COMT inhibitors, selegiline, dopamine agonists, and levodopa and carbidopa.

Surgery may be necessary in rare cases. It was a more common treatment in the past but advance medications have made surgery a last resort or option for patients of Parkinsons disease. Surgeries used for treating Parkinsons disease are thalmotomy, pallidotomy, and deep brain stimulation.

Manufactured by Amazon.ca
Acheson, AB

11784875R00068